HOW TO EAT

Discover the joy of eating well and feel your best every day

Lisa G. Murphy

"How to Eat"

Copyright © 2024 , **Lisa G. Murphy**
All rights reserved.

TABLE OF CONTENT

INTRODUCTION

In a world where mouthwatering, nutritious food satisfies your hunger and stimulates your senses. This book is meant to be your reliable friend in a world where the wealth of dietary knowledge may frequently feel overwhelming, helping you navigate the confusing array of nutritional options with ease, joy, and clarity.

Eating healthily doesn't need restriction or adhering to the newest diet craze. It's about realizing how closely our general health and the food we eat are related. It's about learning how natural, whole foods may improve our health, vitality, and happiness as well as appreciating their colorful flavors and textures.

In "How to Eat," you'll find a wealth of practical advice, that will help you make informed decisions about what goes on your plate. From understanding the essential nutrients your body needs, to mastering the art of meal planning and preparation, this book covers all the bases. You'll also find a collection of mouth-watering recipes that prove healthy eating can be both enjoyable and sustainable.

But this book is more than just a guide; it's an invitation to embrace a new way of thinking about food. Whether you're a seasoned home cook or someone who's just beginning to explore the kitchen, you'll find inspiration and tools to transform your eating habits and, by extension, your life.

Imagine waking up every day feeling energized, clear-headed, and ready to tackle whatever comes your way. Picture yourself savoring meals that not only taste incredible but also nourish your body deeply.

Let's rediscover the joy of eating well and learn how to nourish ourselves in the most profound and pleasurable ways possible

Chapter 1: Cooking with Joy

Welcome to the heart and soul of "How to Eat Well" — the kitchen. In this chapter, we'll explore the concept of cooking with joy, transforming meal preparation from a mundane task into an act of love, creativity, and nourishment. Cooking with joy is about embracing the process, savoring the moments, and appreciating the vibrant, life-giving foods that nature provides.

Many people view cooking as a duty that must be completed quickly at the end of the day. But what if we could change our perspective and saw cooking as a fun and rewarding activity? We enter the kitchen with interest and enthusiasm when we cook with delight. We take pleasure in the meals we prepare and let ourselves experiment with flavors and new ingredients.

Being Present in Preparation

Being present is one of the keys to cooking with delight. We frequently multitask in our fast-paced society, allowing our thoughts to stray even during meal preparation. Try to slow down and give the procedure your whole attention instead. As you chop fresh veggies, feel their texture; smell spices as they sizzle in the pan; and hear the steady rhythmic sounds of cooking. Cooking with mindfulness not only improves your enjoyment of the process but also strengthens your bond with the food you're making.

A Joyful Kitchen Environment

Your kitchen environment plays a significant role in how you feel about cooking. Here are a few tips to create a space that inspires joy:

1. Organization and Cleanliness : A clutter-free, clean kitchen can make cooking more enjoyable. Keep your tools and ingredients organized and easily accessible.

2. Personal Touches : Add elements that make you happy, such as fresh flowers, a favorite cookbook on display, or a playlist of your favorite music.

3. Quality Tools : Invest in a few high-quality kitchen tools. A sharp knife, sturdy cutting board, and reliable cookware can make a big difference in your cooking experience.

Transform your cooking with rituals

You may improve the pleasure of cooking by including rituals into your routine. Perhaps you begin by taking a few deep breaths to focus yourself, putting on your favorite apron, or burning a fragrant candle. These little actions have the power to elevate cooking to a holy and joyous activity.

Cooking joyfully also entails spreading that happiness to other people. Making meals for loved ones and friends can strengthen ties and produce enduring memories. Get family and friends to help you in the kitchen, get kids involved in basic cooking duties, or organize a potluck dinner where everyone brings a dish to share. Cooking and dining together creates a sense of belonging and camaraderie.

Joyful Recipes to Get You Started

To help you embark on your journey of cooking with joy, here are a few simple, delightful recipes:

1. *Rainbow Veggie Stir-Fry*

Ingredients:
- 1 tablespoon olive oil

- 1 red bell pepper, sliced
- 1 yellow bell pepper, sliced
- 1 zucchini, sliced
- 1 carrot, julienned
- 1 cup broccoli florets
- 2 cloves garlic, minced
- 2 tablespoons soy sauce
- 1 tablespoon honey
- 1 teaspoon sesame oil
- Sesame seeds for garnish

Instructions:
1. Heat the olive oil in a large pan over medium heat.
2. Add the garlic and sauté for 1 minute until fragrant.
3. Add all the vegetables and stir-fry for 5-7 minutes until tender but still crisp.
4. Mix the soy sauce, honey, and sesame oil in a small bowl.
5. Pour the sauce over the vegetables and toss to coat.
6. Serve with a sprinkle of sesame seeds.

2. *Lemon Herb Quinoa Salad*

Ingredients:
- 1 cup quinoa, rinsed
- 2 cups water
- 1 cup cherry tomatoes, halved
- 1 cucumber, diced
- 1/4 cup red onion, finely chopped
- 1/4 cup fresh parsley, chopped
- 1/4 cup fresh mint, chopped
- 1/4 cup olive oil
- Juice of 1 lemon
- Salt and pepper to taste

Instructions:
1. Cook the quinoa according to the package instructions and let it cool.
2. In a large bowl, combine the quinoa, cherry tomatoes, cucumber, red onion, parsley, and mint.
3. In a small bowl, whisk together the olive oil, lemon juice, salt, and pepper.
4. Pour the dressing over the salad and toss to combine.

5. Serve chilled or at room temperature.

3. *Berry Bliss Smoothie*

Ingredients:
- 1 cup mixed berries (strawberries,
blueberries, raspberries)
- 1 banana
- 1/2 cup Greek yogurt
- 1/2 cup almond milk
- 1 tablespoon honey
- 1 tablespoon chia seeds

Instructions:
1. Place all ingredients in a blender.
2. Blend until smooth.
3. Pour into a glass and enjoy immediately.

Welcome to a new way of eating well—one
filled with joy, creativity, and nourishment.

Chapter 2: Choosing What to Eat

An essential part of keeping a healthy lifestyle is making food choices. Making the right decisions for your body might be overwhelming with so many alternatives available. You will learn how to choose wholesome meals, comprehend the fundamentals of a balanced diet, and pay attention to your body's needs in this chapter. A well-balanced diet gives your body the vital elements it requires to operate as intended. Here's a quick overview of the primary components:

1. Carbohydrates : The body's main energy source. Focus on complex carbohydrates like whole grains, fruits, and vegetables. These provide sustained energy and are rich in fiber, which aids digestion.

2. Proteins : Crucial for building and repairing tissues. Include a mix of animal and plant-based proteins such as lean meats, fish, eggs, beans, lentils, nuts, and seeds.

3. Fats : Necessary for brain health and energy. Opt for healthy fats found in avocados, nuts, seeds, and olive oil. Limit saturated and trans fats often found in processed foods.

4. Vitamins and Minerals : Essential for various bodily functions. A diverse diet rich in fruits, vegetables, whole grains, and lean proteins typically provides all the vitamins and minerals you need.

5. Water : Vital for overall health, aiding in digestion, nutrient absorption, and temperature regulation. Aim to drink plenty of water throughout the day.

Listening to Your Body

Understanding and listening to your body's signals is key to making informed food choices. Here are some tips:

1. Hunger and Fullness Cues: Learn to recognize when you're genuinely hungry and when you're satisfied. Avoid eating out of boredom, stress, or habit.

2. Cravings : Sometimes, cravings can indicate a deficiency in certain nutrients. For instance, craving chocolate might be a sign of magnesium deficiency. Pay attention to these signals and consider healthier alternatives.

3. Energy Levels : Notice how different foods affect your energy levels. Some foods might make you feel sluggish, while others energize you. Use this information to guide your choices.

4. Digestive Comfort : Pay attention to how your body reacts to different foods. Some people may have intolerances or allergies to certain foods, which can cause discomfort. Choose foods that make you feel good and support your digestive health.

Making Informed Choices

With a basic understanding of nutrition and your body's needs, you can start making informed food choices. Here are some strategies:

1. Read Labels : Understanding food labels can help you make healthier choices. Look for foods with fewer ingredients and avoid those with high amounts of added sugars, sodium, and unhealthy fats.

2. Plan Your Meals : Planning meals in advance can help ensure you have balanced, nutritious options available and reduce the

temptation to opt for unhealthy convenience foods.

3. Incorporate Variety : Eating a variety of foods ensures you get a wide range of nutrients. Try to include different colors and types of fruits and vegetables, various protein sources, and different whole grains in your diet.

4. Prioritize Whole Foods : Whole foods, such as fresh fruits and vegetables, whole grains, lean proteins, and healthy fats, are minimally processed and more nutrient-dense than processed foods.

5. Mindful Eating : Slow down and savor your meals. Mindful eating can enhance your appreciation of food and help you make better choices.

Environmental Impact

Your food choices also have an impact on the environment. Here are some ways to make more sustainable choices:

1. Eat Seasonally : Seasonal produce is often fresher, more nutritious, and has a lower environmental impact because it requires less transportation and storage.

2. Support Local : Buying locally produced foods supports your local economy and reduces the carbon footprint associated with long-distance food transportation.

3. Reduce Food Waste : Plan your meals and portions to minimize waste. Use leftovers creatively and compost food scraps when possible.

4. Choose Plant-Based Options : Incorporating more plant-based meals can reduce your environmental impact, as

plant-based foods generally require fewer resources to produce than animal products.

Choosing what to eat involves

Understanding nutritional basics, listening to your body, making informed decisions, and considering the broader impact of your choices. By focusing on a balanced diet, prioritizing whole foods, and being mindful of your body's signals and the environment, you can create a sustainable, nourishing way of eating that supports your health and well-being.

Chapter 3: The Art of Meal Composition

There is science and art involved in meal preparation. It's all about assembling a meal that pleases the eye, nourishes the body, and is nutritious, balanced, and delights the senses. This chapter will cover meal composition concepts, helpful meal planning advice, and attractive food presentation techniques. A well-planned dinner includes a selection of items to guarantee both sensory satisfaction and nutritional balance. Here are the key components to consider:

1. Balance of Macronutrients : Aim for a mix of carbohydrates, proteins, and fats in each meal. This balance provides sustained energy, supports muscle repair, and keeps you full longer.
   - Carbohydrates : Include whole grains, starchy vegetables, or fruits.

- Proteins : Choose lean meats, fish, eggs, legumes, or plant-based protein sources.
- Fats : Add healthy fats from sources like avocados, nuts, seeds, and olive oil.

2. Variety of Colors and Textures : A visually appealing plate with a variety of colors and textures is more enticing and often more nutritious.
- Colors : Incorporate a rainbow of fruits and vegetables. Each color offers different nutrients and antioxidants.
- Textures : Mix crunchy, creamy, chewy, and soft foods to make the meal more interesting.

3. Portion Control : Understanding portion sizes helps prevent overeating and ensures you get the right amount of nutrients without excess calories.
- Use your plate as a guide: fill half with vegetables, a quarter with protein, and a quarter with whole grains or starchy vegetables.

Practical Tips for Meal Planning

Meal planning is essential for organizing meals efficiently and ensuring you have healthy options available. Here are some strategies:

1. Weekly Planning : Set aside time each week to plan your meals. Decide what you'll eat for breakfast, lunch, dinner, and snacks.
   - Create a shopping list based on your meal plan to avoid impulse buys and ensure you have all necessary ingredients.

2. Batch Cooking : Prepare larger quantities of staple foods (like grains, proteins, and roasted vegetables) that can be used throughout the week.
   - Store these staples in airtight containers for easy assembly into various meals.

3. Prep Ahead : Chop vegetables, marinate proteins, and cook grains ahead of time.

This makes meal assembly quick and easy during busy weekdays.

4. Leftovers : Plan meals that utilize leftovers to minimize waste and save time.
   - For example, a roast chicken can become chicken salad, soup, or tacos later in the week.

Presenting Your Food

The presentation of a meal enhances the dining experience. Here are some tips to elevate the appearance of your dishes:

1. Plating : Use larger plates to give your food space to breathe, and avoid overcrowding. Arrange food attractively, considering balance and symmetry.
   - Place proteins at the center or slightly off-center, with vegetables and grains surrounding them.

2. Garnishing : Fresh herbs, a sprinkle of nuts or seeds, a drizzle of olive oil, or a squeeze of lemon juice can add color and texture to your dishes.

   - Garnishes should complement the flavors and enhance the visual appeal without overwhelming the dish.

3. Layering and Height : Add height to your dishes by layering ingredients or stacking them creatively.

   - For example, layer salads in mason jars or stack roasted vegetables and proteins for a more dynamic presentation.

4. Using Bowls and Plates : Use different types of dishes to suit the meal. Bowls are great for soups, salads, and grain bowls, while plates work well for more structured meals.

   - Experiment with different shapes and sizes to find what works best for each type of food.

Sample Meal Arrangements

Here are some examples to inspire you:

1. Mediterranean Plate

- Protein : Grilled chicken or falafel
- Carbohydrates : Quinoa or couscous
- Vegetables : Roasted bell peppers, zucchini, and cherry tomatoes
- Healthy Fats : Hummus and olives
- Garnish : Fresh parsley and a wedge of lemon

2. Classic Dinner Plate

- Protein : Baked salmon
- Carbohydrates : Sweet potato mash
- Vegetables : Sautéed spinach and roasted Brussels sprouts
- Healthy Fats : Drizzle of olive oil over vegetables
- Garnish : Lemon zest and dill

By planning ahead, incorporating a variety of foods, and paying attention to presentation, you can transform everyday meals into enjoyable culinary experiences. Remember, a well-arranged meal not only looks beautiful but also supports your overall health and well-being.

Chapter 4: Setting the Table

A crucial part of the dining experience is setting the table, which can turn an ordinary meal into a special occasion. It's all about setting up a welcoming environment that makes the food and company even more enjoyable. We'll go over all the fundamentals of table setting in this chapter, including how to place dinnerware and the finer points of creating a cozy atmosphere. Knowing the fundamentals of table setting will help you create a comfortable eating space whether you're hosting a formal or informal dinner by l. Here's a step-by-step guide:

1. Tablecloth and Placemats : Start with a clean tablecloth or placemats to protect your table and add a touch of style. Choose colors and patterns that complement your dining room decor and the occasion.

- For a formal setting, opt for a crisp, white tablecloth. For casual meals, placemats or a patterned tablecloth can add a cozy feel.

2. Dinnerware : Place the dinner plate in the center of each setting. If you're serving multiple courses, layer the salad plate or soup bowl on top of the dinner plate.
   - Charger plates can be used under the dinner plate for a more formal look.

3. Flatware : Arrange the flatware in the order of use, from the outside in. The fork(s) go on the left, and the knife and spoon(s) go on the right.
   - For a formal setting, include a salad fork, dinner fork, dinner knife, soup spoon, and dessert spoon.
   - Ensure the knife blades face inward toward the plate.

4. Glassware : Place the water glass directly above the knife. To the right of the water

glass, position the wine glasses (red and/or white) or other beverage glasses.

   - For formal dinners, you might include a champagne flute or additional glassware as needed.

5. Napkins : Fold the napkin neatly and place it either on the dinner plate or to the left of the forks. Napkin rings can add a decorative touch for special occasions.

6. Bread Plate and Butter Knife : If serving bread, place the bread plate above the forks, with the butter knife laid horizontally across the plate.

Creating a Welcoming Ambiance

The ambiance of your dining area can significantly enhance the dining experience. Here are some tips to create a warm and inviting atmosphere:

1. Lighting : Adjust the lighting to suit the occasion. Soft, warm lighting creates an intimate and cozy atmosphere. Candles are perfect for adding a romantic touch or for special dinners.
   - Avoid harsh overhead lights. Consider using dimmers, table lamps, or fairy lights to create a softer glow.

2. Centerpieces : A beautiful centerpiece adds charm to the table. Fresh flowers, potted plants, or a bowl of seasonal fruits can serve as an attractive focal point.
   - Ensure the centerpiece is not too tall or obstructive, allowing guests to see and converse with each other easily.

3. Music : Background music can enhance the dining experience. Choose a playlist that complements the mood of your meal—soft jazz, classical, or acoustic tunes are great options for a relaxed atmosphere.

- Keep the volume low enough to allow for conversation without needing to raise voices.

4. Personal Touches : Add personal touches to make the table setting unique and special. This could include place cards with guests' names, themed decorations, or small, thoughtful details like handwritten menus.
   - Personal touches show your guests that you've put thought and care into their dining experience.

Table Etiquette for Hosts and Guests

Good table etiquette contributes to a pleasant dining experience. Here are some etiquette tips for both hosts and guests:

1. For Hosts :
   - Welcome Guests : Greet your guests warmly and make them feel at home.

- Serve Promptly : Try to serve food promptly to avoid long waits between courses.
- Engage : Engage with your guests, ensuring everyone is included in the conversation.
- Attentiveness : Pay attention to your guests' needs, such as refilling drinks and clearing plates.

2. For Guests :
- Arrive on Time : Punctuality shows respect for the host's efforts.
- RSVP : Let the host know if you can attend and inform them of any dietary restrictions in advance.
- Politeness : Use polite manners, such as saying please and thank you, and wait for everyone to be served before starting to eat.
- Engagement : Engage in conversation and show appreciation for the meal and effort put in by the host.

Sample Table Settings

Here are examples of different table settings to inspire you:

1. Casual Family Dinner

- Tablecloth/Placemats : Colorful placemats
- Dinnerware : Simple dinner plates with coordinating salad plates
- Flatware : Basic fork, knife, and spoon
- Glassware : Water glass and one wine glass
- Napkins : Folded cloth napkins in a simple holder
- Centerpiece : A small vase of fresh flowers or a bowl of fruits

2. Formal Dinner Party

- Tablecloth/Placemats: Elegant white tablecloth
- Dinnerware : Charger plates, dinner plates, salad plates, and soup bowls

- Flatware : Full set including salad fork, dinner fork, knife, soup spoon, and dessert spoon
- Glassware : Water glass, red wine glass, white wine glass, and champagne flute
- Napkins : Cloth napkins with napkin rings
- Centerpiece : Low floral arrangement or candles

3. Themed Celebration

- Tablecloth/Placemats : Themed tablecloth (e.g., holiday, seasonal)
- Dinnerware : Coordinated themed plates and bowls
- Flatware : Standard set with decorative handles
- Glassware : Fun, themed glasses or regular glassware with themed markers
- Napkins : Themed or color-coordinated napkins
- Centerpiece : Themed decorations, such as holiday ornaments or seasonal items

More than merely setting out dishes and silverware, setting the table involves creating a cozy and welcoming environment where people may enjoy their meals to the utmost. You and your guests can enjoy a better dining experience if you know how to arrange the table, add a personal touch, and create a cozy atmosphere. Keep in mind that a carefully arranged table fosters conversation and creates an atmosphere for showcasing your culinary delights.

Chapter 5: Sitting While You Eat

Eating has become a hurried activity in our fast-paced world, typically crammed in between other chores. But eating may become more than just a necessity when you sit down to eat; it can become a mindful and pleasurable experience. This chapter examines the value of eating in a seated position, the advantages of mindful eating, and useful advice for establishing a more contented and unwinding lunchtime habit.

Sitting down to eat is about more than just physical posture; it's a practice that can significantly impact your overall health and well-being. Here's why it matters:

1. Digestive Health: Sitting down allows your body to relax and focus on digestion. Eating on the go or standing can lead to indigestion, bloating, and discomfort

because your body is in a more active state, which can impede the digestive process.

2. Mindful Eating : When you sit down to eat, you're more likely to pay attention to your food, savor each bite, and recognize your body's hunger and fullness cues. This mindfulness can help prevent overeating and promote a healthier relationship with food.

3. Social Connection : Shared meals around a table foster social interaction and connection. Sitting down to eat with family or friends provides an opportunity to bond, share stories, and create memories.

4. Stress Reduction : Taking a break to sit and enjoy your meal can reduce stress levels. It allows you to step away from the busyness of the day, providing a moment of calm and relaxation.

The Benefits of Mindful Eating

Mindful eating involves paying full attention to the experience of eating and drinking, both inside and outside the body. The benefits of this practice are numerous:

1. Improved Digestion : Mindful eating encourages slower eating, which can improve digestion and nutrient absorption. Chewing thoroughly and taking time between bites helps your body process food more effectively.

2. Better Portion Control : By paying attention to hunger and fullness signals, you're less likely to overeat. Mindful eaters often find they can enjoy smaller portions and feel satisfied.

3. Enhanced Enjoyment : Focusing on the flavors, textures, and aromas of your food enhances the eating experience, making meals more pleasurable and satisfying.

4. Emotional Regulation : Mindful eating
can help break the cycle of emotional eating.
By being present with your food, you're
more aware of why you're eating and can
make more conscious choices.

**Practical Tips for Sitting and Eating
Mindfully**

Integrating the practice of sitting and eating
mindfully into your daily routine can be
simple with these practical tips:

1. Create a Pleasant Eating Environment :
Set up a dedicated eating area that's
comfortable and free from distractions. This
can be a dining table, a cozy nook, or even a
spot outside when the weather is nice.
   - Ensure the area is clean and tidy, which
can enhance the overall experience.

2. Set Aside Time for Meals: Schedule
regular meal times and give yourself enough

time to sit and enjoy your food without
rushing.
   - Treat mealtime as an important
appointment with yourself.

3. Minimize Distractions: Turn off the TV,
put away your phone, and focus on the meal
in front of you. Reducing distractions helps
you tune into the eating experience.
   - If you're eating with others, engage in
conversation rather than scrolling through
devices.

4. Start with Deep Breaths : Before you
begin eating, take a few deep breaths to
center yourself. This helps signal to your
body that it's time to relax and focus on the
meal.
   - Deep breathing can also help reduce
stress and improve digestion.

5. Chew Thoroughly ikojioc: Chewing each
bite thoroughly not only aids digestion but

also allows you to fully experience the flavors and textures of your food.

  - Aim to chew each bite at least 20-30 times before swallowing.

6. Pause Between Bites : Put your fork down between bites to slow down your eating pace. This gives your body time to register fullness and enhances mindful eating.

  - Sipping water between bites can also help you eat more slowly.

7. Appreciate Your Food : Take a moment to appreciate the food you're about to eat. Consider where it came from, the effort involved in preparing it, and the nourishment it provides.

  - Expressing gratitude can enhance your overall eating experience.

8. Listen to Your Body : Pay attention to your body's hunger and fullness cues. Eat when you're hungry and stop when you're

satisfied, not necessarily when your plate is clean.

 - This practice helps prevent overeating and promotes a healthy relationship with food.

Overcoming Challenges

Integrating the practice of sitting and eating mindfully can come with challenges, especially in a busy lifestyle. Here are some common obstacles and ways to overcome them:

1. Time Constraints : If you're pressed for time, try to at least sit down for a short period. Even a few minutes of focused eating is better than none.

 - Meal prepping and planning can help create more time for mindful eating.

2. Habits and Routines : Breaking the habit of eating on the go or in front of screens can be difficult. Start by setting small,

achievable goals, like dedicating one meal a day to mindful eating.

   - Gradually increase the number of mindful meals as you become more comfortable with the practice.

3. Social Dynamics : In social settings, it can be challenging to stay mindful. Engage in conversations that revolve around the meal and the experience of eating to help keep your focus.

   - Encourage mindful eating practices among family and friends to create a supportive environment.

Sitting while you eat is a simple yet powerful practice that can enhance your physical and emotional well-being. By making mealtime a mindful, seated experience, you can improve digestion, enjoy your food more fully, and foster deeper connections with those around you. Embrace the practice of sitting down to eat as a way to nourish not just your body, but also your mind and spirit.

Chapter 6: The Right Amount

Understanding how much food your body needs is crucial for maintaining a healthy weight and overall well-being. In a world where portion sizes have grown significantly, it can be challenging to gauge what constitutes an appropriate amount. This chapter explores how to determine the right portion sizes, listen to your body's hunger and fullness cues, and make mindful eating decisions.

Understanding Portion Sizes

Portion sizes have a direct impact on your caloric intake and nutritional balance. Here's how to navigate and understand them:

1. Serving Size vs. Portion Size :
   - Serving Size : This is a standardized amount of food, often used on nutrition

labels to help you understand the nutritional content of that specific amount.

- Portion Size : This is the amount of food you choose to eat in one sitting, which may be more or less than the serving size.

2. Visual Cues : Use everyday objects to help visualize appropriate portion sizes:

- Meat or Protein : A serving size is roughly the size of a deck of cards or the palm of your hand.

- Vegetables and Fruits : A serving is about the size of your fist.

- Grains and Starchy Vegetables : A serving is approximately the size of a tennis ball or a cupped hand.

- Fats and Oils : A serving size is about the size of your thumb.

3. Plate Method : Divide your plate to help balance your meal:

- Half the Plate : Fill with vegetables and fruits.

- One-Quarter of the Plate : Fill with lean protein sources.
- One-Quarter of the Plate : Fill with whole grains or starchy vegetables.

Listening to Your Body's Cues

Your body naturally signals when it needs food and when it has had enough. Learning to recognize these signals can prevent overeating and promote a healthier relationship with food.

1. Hunger Cues : Physical signs that you need to eat include a growling stomach, low energy, and difficulty concentrating. Emotional hunger, such as eating out of boredom or stress, can be identified by cravings for specific comfort foods rather than general hunger.
- Eat when you feel physical hunger rather than waiting until you're ravenous to avoid overeating.

2. Fullness Cues : Signs of fullness include feeling satisfied, no longer having a desire to eat, and a sense of comfort in your stomach. It takes about 20 minutes for your brain to register fullness, so eating slowly can help you tune in to these signals.
   - Stop eating when you feel satisfied, not stuffed. Eating slowly and pausing between bites can help you recognize when you've had enough.

3. Mindful Eating Practices :
   - Slow Down : Take your time to chew and savor each bite.
   - Focus on Food : Minimize distractions such as TV or smartphones.
   - Reflect on Hunger : Before reaching for food, ask yourself if you are truly hungry or if there's another emotion driving the desire to eat.

Practical Strategies for Determining How Much is Enough

Applying practical strategies can help you better manage portion sizes and ensure you're eating the right amount for your needs.

1. Start with Smaller Portions : Begin with smaller servings and allow yourself to have more if you're still hungry. This helps prevent overeating and gives you better control over your intake.
   - Use smaller plates and bowls to naturally limit portion sizes.

2. Measure and Weigh : Occasionally measure or weigh your food to get a better understanding of portion sizes. This can be particularly helpful with calorie-dense foods like nuts, oils, and grains.
   - Keep measuring cups and a food scale handy in the kitchen.

3. Mindful Snacking : When snacking, portion out a serving into a bowl rather than eating directly from the package. This helps you keep track of how much you're consuming.
   - Choose snacks that are nutrient-dense and satisfying, such as fruits, vegetables, nuts, or yogurt.

4. Balanced Meals : Ensure each meal includes a balance of macronutrients (carbohydrates, proteins, and fats) to keep you satisfied and prevent overeating.
   - Incorporate fiber-rich foods and healthy fats to help you feel fuller longer.

Overcoming Portion Distortion

Portion distortion refers to the perception that large portions are the norm, which can lead to overeating. Here's how to overcome it:

1. Awareness : Educate yourself about standard portion sizes and compare them to what you typically consume. This awareness can help you make more informed choices.
   - Refer to nutrition labels and serving size guides for accurate information.

2. Restaurant Portions : Restaurant portions are often much larger than necessary. Consider sharing a dish, asking for a half-portion, or taking part of your meal home.
   - Practice portion control even when dining out by splitting meals or choosing appetizers as main courses.

3. Mindful Grocery Shopping : Buy single-serving packages or portion out larger packages into smaller, individual servings. This can help prevent the temptation to overeat.
   - Plan your meals and snacks in advance to avoid impulse buying and overconsumption.

By practicing these strategies, you can better manage your food intake, maintain a healthy weight, and enjoy a more balanced and fulfilling relationship with food. Remember, eating the right amount isn't about restriction—it's about finding the balance that works best for your body and lifestyle.

Chapter 7: Eating with Attention

In today's fast-paced world, eating has become an automatic activity often done on the go, in front of screens, or amidst numerous distractions. Mindful eating is a powerful practice that can transform your relationship with food, enhance your dining experience, and improve your overall health. This chapter delves into the principles of mindful eating, its benefits, and practical ways to incorporate it into your daily life.

What is Mindful Eating?

Mindful eating is the practice of being fully present during meals, paying attention to the sensory experience of eating, and recognizing physical hunger and satiety cues. It involves savoring food, appreciating its flavors and textures, and understanding the emotional and physical sensations associated with eating.

Mindful eating is based on several core principles:

1. Awareness : Being conscious of what you're eating, how you're eating, and why you're eating. This includes noticing the taste, texture, and smell of your food, as well as your body's hunger and fullness signals.

2. Non-Judgment : Approaching eating without judgment, guilt, or anxiety. It's about enjoying food and the eating experience without labeling foods as "good" or "bad."

3. Presence : Staying present in the moment, focusing solely on the act of eating. This means eliminating distractions such as TV, smartphones, or multitasking during meals.

4. Savoring : Taking the time to savor each bite, appreciating the effort that went into preparing the meal, and the journey the food took to reach your plate.

Benefits of Mindful Eating

Practicing mindful eating offers numerous benefits for your physical, mental, and emotional well-being:

1. Improved Digestion : Eating slowly and mindfully can enhance digestion by allowing your body to process food more efficiently. Chewing thoroughly and taking time between bites helps break down food properly.

2. Better Weight Management : Mindful eating can help prevent overeating and support healthy weight management. By paying attention to hunger and fullness cues, you're less likely to consume excess calories.

3. Enhanced Enjoyment : Mindful eating increases the enjoyment of food. By focusing on the sensory experience, you can derive more pleasure from each meal and appreciate the flavors and textures more fully.

4. Reduced Emotional Eating : Becoming aware of the emotional triggers for eating can help you make more conscious food choices. Mindful eating can reduce reliance on food for comfort and address underlying emotional needs in healthier ways.

5. Balanced Relationship with Food : Mindful eating promotes a healthier relationship with food by fostering a non-judgmental approach. It encourages self-compassion and reduces feelings of guilt or shame associated with eating.

Practical Strategies for Mindful Eating

Incorporating mindful eating into your daily routine can be simple with these practical strategies:

1. Set the Scene : Create a calm and inviting eating environment. Set the table, eliminate distractions, and make your dining space comfortable and aesthetically pleasing.

2. Pause Before Eating : Take a moment to pause and take a few deep breaths before starting your meal. This helps center your mind and body, preparing you to focus on the eating experience.

3. Engage Your Senses : Notice the colors, textures, and aromas of your food. Pay attention to the flavors and how they change as you chew. Engage all your senses to fully experience the meal.

4. Chew Thoroughly : Chewing your food thoroughly aids digestion and allows you to savor the flavors. Aim to chew each bite at least 20-30 times before swallowing.

5. Eat Slowly : Slow down your eating pace by putting your fork down between bites and taking smaller bites. This gives your body time to register fullness and enhances the enjoyment of your meal.

6. Listen to Your Body : Pay attention to your body's hunger and fullness cues. Eat when you're hungry and stop when you're satisfied, not necessarily when your plate is clean.

7. Reflect on Your Meal : After eating, take a moment to reflect on the meal. Consider how the food made you feel, the flavors you enjoyed, and any sensations of hunger or fullness.

Overcoming Common Challenges

Mindful eating can be challenging, especially in a busy lifestyle. Here are some common obstacles and ways to overcome them:

1. Distractions : It can be difficult to eliminate distractions, but small steps can make a big difference. Start by dedicating at least one meal a day to mindful eating, gradually increasing as you become more comfortable.

2. Time Constraints : If you're short on time, focus on making at least part of your meal mindful. Even a few minutes of focused eating can have positive effects. Meal prepping can also help create more time for mindful eating.

3. Emotional Eating : Mindful eating can help address emotional eating by increasing awareness of emotional triggers. Practice

self-compassion and seek alternative ways to cope with emotions, such as talking to a friend or engaging in a hobby.

4. Habitual Eating : Breaking old habits takes time. Be patient with yourself and start small. Celebrate your successes and learn from setbacks.

Chapter 8: Eat gently

In a society that often equates speed with efficiency, the idea of slowing down can seem counterintuitive. However, when it comes to eating, taking your time is essential for both physical health and emotional well-being. This chapter explores the benefits of slowing down during meals, the science behind why it works, and practical tips for integrating a slower pace into your eating habits.

Importance of Slowing Down

Eating slowly can significantly improve the quality of your meals and your overall health. Here are some reasons why it's beneficial to slow down:

1. Better Digestion : When you eat slowly, you chew your food more thoroughly, which aids in the initial stages of digestion. This allows your stomach to break down food

more efficiently and can help prevent digestive issues such as bloating and indigestion.

2. Enhanced Satiety : It takes about 20 minutes for your brain to register that your stomach is full. Eating slowly gives your body the time it needs to signal satiety, which can prevent overeating and help maintain a healthy weight.

3. Increased Enjoyment : Slowing down allows you to savor the flavors, textures, and aromas of your food. This can enhance your overall eating experience and lead to greater satisfaction with your meals.

4. Mindful Eating : Eating at a slower pace encourages mindfulness. It helps you stay present and focused on the act of eating, making you more aware of your hunger and fullness cues.

5. Reduced Stress : Taking the time to eat slowly can serve as a break in your day, providing a moment of calm and relaxation. This can help reduce stress and improve your mental well-being.

The Science Behind Eating Slowly

Scientific research supports the benefits of eating at a slower pace. Studies have shown that people who eat quickly are more likely to consume more calories and gain weight compared to those who eat slowly. Here's why:

1. Hormonal Responses : Eating slowly can positively influence the hormones that regulate hunger and fullness. Hormones like ghrelin (which stimulates appetite) and leptin (which signals satiety) work more effectively when you give your body time to process the food.

2. Metabolic Rate : Eating slowly can help maintain a steady metabolic rate. Rapid eating can cause spikes in blood sugar levels, leading to energy crashes and increased hunger later on.

3. Portion Control : Slower eating promotes better portion control. When you take your time, you're more likely to stop eating when you're full, rather than when your plate is empty.

Practical Tips for Slowing Down

Slowing down during meals may require a shift in habits and mindset. Here are some practical tips to help you eat more slowly:

1. Chew Thoroughly : Aim to chew each bite at least 20-30 times. This not only aids digestion but also allows you to fully appreciate the flavors and textures of your food.

- Focus on the act of chewing and notice how the food changes in your mouth.

2. Put Down Your Utensils : Place your fork or spoon down between bites. This simple act can help you slow your pace and give your body time to signal fullness.
   - Take a sip of water or engage in conversation during these pauses.

3. Take Smaller Bites : Cutting your food into smaller pieces and taking smaller bites can help you eat more slowly and mindfully.
   - Appreciate each bite and notice the different tastes and sensations.

4. Set a Timer : Use a timer to pace your meals. Start with a goal of extending your meal time by 5-10 minutes and gradually increase as you get more comfortable.
   - Aim for meals to last at least 20-30 minutes.

5. Engage Your Senses : Focus on the sensory experience of eating. Notice the colors, smells, and textures of your food. This can enhance your enjoyment and encourage a slower pace.
   - Engage all your senses to fully experience the meal.

6. Create a Calm Eating Environment : Minimize distractions by turning off the TV, putting away your phone, and creating a peaceful dining space. This helps you focus on your meal and eat more slowly.
   - Choose a comfortable and inviting space for your meals.

7. Practice Gratitude : Take a moment before eating to express gratitude for your food. This can help you approach your meal with a sense of appreciation and mindfulness.
   - Reflect on the journey of the food from farm to table.

Overcoming Challenges to Slowing Down

Slowing down can be challenging, especially if you're accustomed to eating quickly. Here are some common obstacles and ways to overcome them:

1. Busy Schedules : If you're short on time, even a few minutes of mindful eating can make a difference. Start with one meal a day and gradually increase as you become more comfortable.
   - Meal prepping can also create more time for slower, mindful eating.

2. Habitual Fast Eating : Breaking the habit of eating quickly takes time. Be patient with yourself and start with small, achievable goals.
   - Celebrate your progress and learn from setbacks.

3. Social Pressures : In social settings, it can be tempting to eat quickly to keep pace with others. Focus on enjoying the company and conversation, and set your own pace.
   - Encourage mindful eating practices among friends and family.

4. Emotional Eating : If you tend to eat quickly when stressed or emotional, find alternative ways to cope with your feelings. Practice mindfulness and stress-reduction techniques such as deep breathing or meditation.
   - Seek support from friends, family, or a therapist if needed.

Embrace the practice of slowing down as a way to nourish your body, mind, and spirit, and discover the joy and satisfaction of truly savoring each meal.

Chapter 9: Good Appetite

A healthy appetite is a sign of a well-functioning body and a positive relationship with food. However, understanding what constitutes a "good appetite" can be nuanced, as it varies from person to person based on individual needs, lifestyle, and health conditions. In this chapter, we explore the concept of a good appetite, the factors that influence it, and how to maintain a healthy and balanced appetite through mindful practices and lifestyle adjustments.

Understanding a Good Appetite

A good appetite is an indication that your body's metabolism and digestive system are working harmoniously. It reflects your body's natural demand for energy and nutrients. Here are some characteristics of a healthy appetite:

1. Regular Hunger Signals : Feeling hungry at regular intervals throughout the day, typically every 3-4 hours, indicates a healthy appetite.

2. Satisfaction After Eating : Eating should lead to a feeling of satisfaction and satiety without feeling overly full or still hungry.

3. Cravings for Nutrient-Dense Foods : A healthy appetite often includes cravings for a variety of foods, including fruits, vegetables, proteins, and whole grains.

4. Flexibility : Being able to adapt your appetite to different situations, such as eating more during periods of physical activity or less when sedentary.

Factors Influencing Appetite

Several factors can influence your appetite, including physiological, psychological, and environmental elements:

1. Physiological Factors : Hormones such as ghrelin (which stimulates hunger) and

leptin (which signals satiety) play crucial roles in regulating appetite. Blood sugar levels, metabolic rate, and overall health also affect hunger and fullness cues.

2. Psychological Factors : Stress, anxiety, depression, and emotional states can significantly impact appetite. Emotional eating or loss of appetite can be responses to psychological conditions.

3. Environmental Factors : Availability of food, portion sizes, social settings, and cultural norms can influence how much and what you eat.

4. Lifestyle Factors : Physical activity levels, sleep patterns, and daily routines can affect your appetite. Regular exercise typically enhances appetite, while poor sleep can disrupt hunger hormones.

Maintaining a Healthy Appetite

Balancing your appetite involves listening to your body, making mindful food choices, and adopting healthy lifestyle habits. Here are some strategies to help maintain a good appetite:

1. Eat Balanced Meals : Ensure your meals contain a balance of macronutrients—carbohydrates, proteins, and fats—along with fiber. This helps stabilize blood sugar levels and promotes sustained energy and satiety.
   - Include a variety of colorful fruits and vegetables, lean proteins, whole grains, and healthy fats in your diet.

2. Stay Hydrated : Dehydration can sometimes be mistaken for hunger. Drinking adequate water throughout the day can help regulate your appetite.
   - Aim for at least 8 cups of water daily, and more if you're physically active or in a hot climate.

3. Regular Physical Activity : Exercise boosts metabolism and can help regulate hunger

and fullness cues. Aim for a mix of cardio, strength training, and flexibility exercises.
   - Find activities you enjoy, such as walking, swimming, or yoga, to stay consistent.

4. Mindful Eating : Practice mindful eating by paying attention to hunger and fullness cues, eating slowly, and savoring each bite. This can help you tune in to your body's needs and prevent overeating.
   - Avoid distractions such as TV or smartphones during meals to focus on the eating experience.

5. Regular Meal Times : Eating at consistent times each day helps regulate your body's hunger signals and can improve digestion.
   - Try to have breakfast, lunch, and dinner around the same times daily, with healthy snacks in between if needed.

6. Healthy Snacking : Choose nutrient-dense snacks such as nuts, fruits, vegetables, or

yogurt to keep your energy levels stable between meals.
  - Avoid processed snacks high in sugar and unhealthy fats, which can lead to energy crashes and increased hunger.

7. Manage Stress : Chronic stress can disrupt appetite regulation. Incorporate stress-reduction techniques such as meditation, deep breathing exercises, or hobbies that you enjoy.
  - Practice self-care and seek support if stress becomes overwhelming.

8. Get Adequate Sleep : Poor sleep can affect hunger hormones and lead to increased appetite and cravings for unhealthy foods. Aim for 7-9 hours of quality sleep each night.
  - Establish a regular sleep routine and create a restful sleep environment.

Recognizing Changes in Appetite

It's essential to be aware of significant changes in your appetite, as they can indicate underlying health issues. Here are some signs to watch for:

1. Sudden Increase in Appetite : While occasional increases in hunger can be normal, a sudden and persistent increase may require attention. Potential causes include hormonal imbalances, hyperthyroidism, or stress.
   - Monitor your eating patterns and consult a healthcare professional if the increase is unexplained.

2. Loss of Appetite : A significant and sustained decrease in appetite can be concerning and may indicate conditions such as depression, anxiety, or gastrointestinal issues.
   - Seek medical advice if you experience a prolonged lack of interest in food.

3. Changes Due to Medication : Some medications can affect appetite as a side effect. If you notice changes after starting a new medication, consult your doctor for guidance.

   - Discuss alternative medications or dosage adjustments with your healthcare provider if needed.

A good appetite is a cornerstone of a healthy, balanced lifestyle. By understanding the factors that influence your appetite and adopting mindful and healthy eating practices, you can maintain a positive relationship with food. Listening to your body's signals, eating a varied and nutrient-dense diet, staying hydrated, managing stress, and ensuring adequate sleep are all key components of nurturing a healthy appetite. Embrace these practices to enjoy your meals fully, maintain your well-being, and support your overall health.

References

In writing this book, numerous sources have been consulted to provide accurate, comprehensive, and insightful information on eating well. Below are the references, which include scientific studies, books, and reputable online resources that have contributed to the content.

Books

1. Brown, D. (2018). *The Joy of Cooking*. New York: Scribner.
2. Pollan, M. (2008). *In Defense of Food: An Eater's Manifesto*. New York: Penguin Press.
3. Satter, E. (2008). *Secrets of Feeding a Healthy Family*. Madison: Kelcy Press.
4. Wansink, B. (2010). *Mindless Eating: Why We Eat More Than We Think*. New York: Bantam Books.

Scientific Journals

1. Flint, A., Raben, A., Blundell, J. E., & Astrup, A. (2000). Reproducibility, power and validity of visual analogue scales in assessment of appetite sensations in single test meal studies. *International Journal of Obesity*, 24(1), 38-48.
2. Rolls, B. J., Roe, L. S., & Meengs, J. S. (2007). The effect of large portion sizes on energy intake is sustained for 11 days. *Obesity*, 15(6), 1535-1543.
3. Schachter, S. (1971). Some extraordinary facts about obese humans and rats. *American Psychologist*, 26(2), 129-144.

Online Resources

1. Harvard T.H. Chan School of Public Health. (2021). *The Nutrition Source: Healthy Eating Plate*. Retrieved from [https://www.hsph.harvard.edu/nutritionsource/healthy-eating-plate/](https://www.hs

ph.harvard.edu/nutritionsource/healthy-eat
ing-plate/)
2. Mayo Clinic. (2020). *Mindful Eating:
Savor the Flavor*. Retrieved from
[https://www.mayoclinic.org/healthy-lifesty
le/nutrition-and-healthy-eating/in-depth/m
indful-eating/art-20267144](https://www.
mayoclinic.org/healthy-lifestyle/nutrition-a
nd-healthy-eating/in-depth/mindful-eating
/art-20267144)
3. National Institute of Diabetes and
Digestive and Kidney Diseases. (2017).
Digestive Diseases: What Is Digestion?.
Retrieved from
[https://www.niddk.nih.gov/health-informa
tion/digestive-diseases/digestion](https://
www.niddk.nih.gov/health-information/dig
estive-diseases/digestion)
4. NHS. (2019). *Portion Sizes: How to
Portion Your Food*. Retrieved from
[https://www.nhs.uk/live-well/eat-well/por
tion-size-tips/](https://www.nhs.uk/live-we
ll/eat-well/portion-size-tips/)

Additional Readings

1. Bauer, J., & Liou, D. (2015). Nutrition Counseling and Education Skill Development. Belmont: Cengage Learning.
2. Bratman, S., & Knight, D. (2000). Health Food Junkies: Orthorexia Nervosa: Overcoming the Obsession with Healthful Eating. New York: Broadway Books.

ISBN 9798329439946

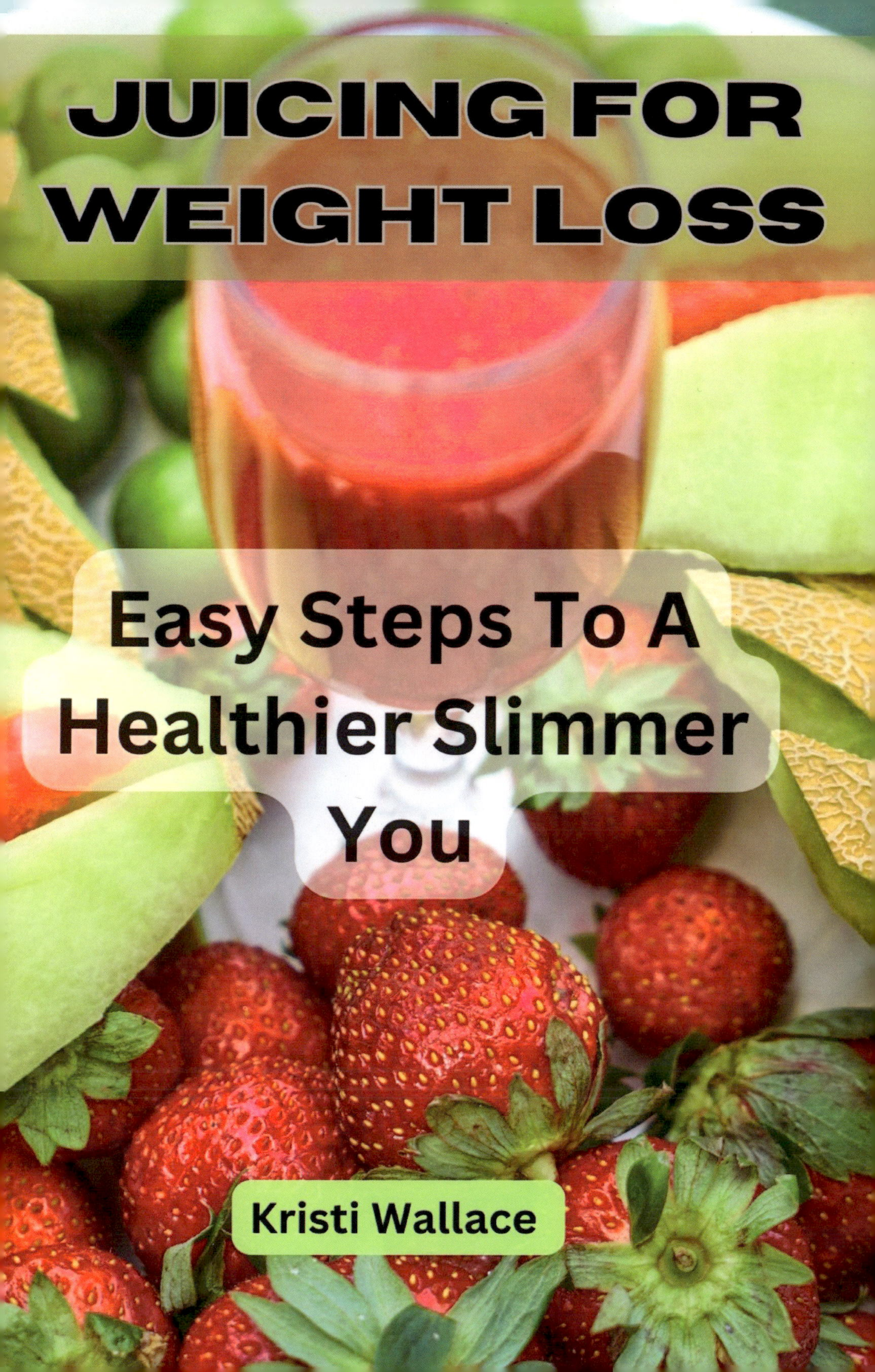

JUICING FOR WEIGHT LOSS
Easy Steps To A Healthier Slimmer You
Kristi Wallace